Herbalism for beginners

This book is an essential guide about the use and formation of herbal remedies and self-medication. Learn the most common medicinal herbs you can grow at home. "Catherine White"

- CHAPTER1: INTRODUCTION ABOUT HERBALISM

- CHAPTER2: HISTORY OF HERBALISM AND HERBAL MEDICINE

- CHAPTER3: WHY TO CHOOSE HERBALISM OVER OTHER SCHOOL OF THOUGHTS

- CHAPTER4: DETAILS ABOUT PLANTS USED IN HERBALISM

- CHAPTER5: RECIPES FOR EVERYDAY HEALTH

- CHAPTER6: HERBS AS HEALING REMEDIES

Contents

CHAPTER 1: INTRODUCTION ABOUT HERBALISM...............8

Herbalism: 8

Specific terminologies related to herbalism: 11

Different types of herbalism: 13

Herbalism versus different medical systems: 14

Evaluation of herbs for medical uses:...............17

Organoleptic analysis: 17

Microscopic analysis: 17

Physical analysis: 18

Chemical analysis: 18

Biological analysis:...............18

CHAPTER 2: HISTORY OF HERBALISM AND HERBAL MEDICINE:...............20

Traditional Indian medicine: 21

Traditional Chinese medicine:...............22

Traditional Egyptian medicine: 23

Roman and Greek era of medicine: 23

Traditional Islamic medicine: 24

American/western traditional medicine:...............24

CHAPTER 3: WHY TO CHOOSE HERBALISM OVER OTHER SCHOOL OF THOUGHTS...............29

CHAPTER 4: DETAILS ABOUT CLASSIFICATION OF PLANTS USED IN HERBALISM 33

Classification on the basis of different characteristics: 33

In alphabetical order: 34

On the basis of taxonomy: 34

On the basis of morphology: 34

Therapeutic purposes: 35

Action-based classification: 35

According to systems of the body: 35

Classification on the basis of medical systems: 35

Biochemical system of classification: 35

Biogenetic type of classification: 36

Geographical classification: 36

CHAPTER 5: HERBS AS HEALING REMEDIES 38

Acerola...38

Alpha-lipoic acid: 40

Amla or Indian berry: 41

Ashwagandha: 42

Astragalus 43

Bacopa 45

Bilberry 48

Cordyceps 50

Devil's Club...51

Elderberry 53

Eleuthero..55

Details:...55

Epimedium: 56

Eurycoma 59

Ginger: 61

Ginseng 67

Green tea: 70

Oat seed: 72

CHAPTER 6: RECIPES FOR EVERYDAY HEALTH 75

Quality control and assessment of herbs: 76

Guidelines about dosing: 80

Recipies and ways of preparation for herbal medicine: 82

Teas:...82

Decoctions 84

Popsicles: 85

Ice cubes: 85

Baths: 85

Breast milk:..86

Washcloths: 87

Compresses:...88

Poultices: 88

Tinctures 90

Summary:..92

CHAPTER 1: INTRODUCTION ABOUT HERBALISM

Herbalism:

Herbalism is by far the most historical type of medical treatment strategy implemented by nearly every era of the human race and in every country of the world. Herbalism is the use of herbs for therapeutic purposes and poses a deep relationship between man and plant. It is widely practiced by every human culture, race, or religion. Herbalism is the most natural type of medical treatment in which herbs are grown and used to reduce the risks associated with herbs. A wide variety of different methods are implicated in using herbs for therapeutic purposes. Tinctures, solutions, grains, oils, and many other forms of herbs are used as a medication to treat nearly every system of the human body.

A herbalist is a person who grows, prepares, and uses herbs to treat the illnesses related to the human mind, body, and spirit. Herbalism has its basis on holistic pharma in which physical, emotional, and spiritual aspects of the human body are treated instead of just treating the cause. It is very different than homeopathy, allopathy (modern medicine), and other types of medical schools in treating human illnesses.

The herbalism is actually the pythotherapy in medical terminology in which plants are used to the mind, body, and spirit of a human being. It is a branch of holistic medicine in which specific herbs are used to treat multiple illnesses and conditions. It is comprised of the principle and practice of art and medicine to create a system of treatment. Nearly any condition which can be treated by allopath, homeopathy or other medicine systems can also be treated by herbal medicine. The benefits hidden in plants can affect the human physiological responses, and thus, any disturbances in them can also be treated by using plants as a medicine. Holistic medicine is evolving these days, and its roots are getting stronger day by day. Nearly every country of the world is using a holistic approach to medicine in every medical field. This shift of paradigm is not new to humankind, and it has historical grounds as well.

WHO is the official body which is responsible for defining the standard definitions related to medical and health. The definition of WHO about health involves the spiritual and mental aspects along with the physical integration of a human being, and it forces the practitioner to treat the human as a whole. A system of self-healing strategy is also an equally important concept in pythotherapy and holistic medicine. Hippocratic Oath also guides the herbalist to use strategies to treat human-being as a whole. A medical practitioner can be a Doctor or herbal medicine, osteopath, physician, or a qualified nurse who can use alternative therapies that are in the domain of holistic medicine and have a strong research background. It is of great importance to discuss the regulations and roles of medical herbalism practitioners who can use a holistic approach to treat patients. Nature greatly assists the philosophy and practice of a medical herbalism expert. The healing strategy used by a medical herbalist is called ecological healing because it uses plants and the ecological environment for healing of a condition.

The high strength of herbalism expert is the integration of traditional philosophies of healing with modern day scope of practice. Medical herbalism is very simple and highly complex at the same time. It is merely that a patient can get the maximum benefit of a weed by just growing it in his/her backyard and chewing it or drinking the dissolved solution. The complexities lie in the fundamental biochemical and pharmacological aspects of a herb using as a treatment of choice. The self-healing strategy used by a medical herbalist is to introduce a patient about a specific herb and providing him knowledge of proper uses and benefits of that specific herb. He/she makes the patient eligible to grow his/her own weed or herb and thus, provides a higher degree of autonomy to the patient. From a seed to a complete plant, a patient seeks close attachment with the growth of that plant, and thus, the benefits on the mind, body, and spirit of a patient introduced by the plant are many folds. In medical herbalism practice, a properly educated patient works in close coordination with a plant that not only cures his/her physical illnesses but also helps in experience a whole new life, from a seed to a full-grown plant.

A plant is a living entity that breaths, exchanges gases, grows while consuming the nutrition, and dies when depletion of nutrients occurs. Life and death are very similar as experienced by the human. So, this experience is highly crucial for a herbalist to know the basic principles of personal healing. An educated patient who experiences this phenomenon by himself can understand the art of living in a broader vision, and a much deeper attachment with the plant can also be obtained. This fantastic interaction affects the physiological responses occurring in mind, body, and spirit of humans, and thus, complete health in the context of physical, emotional, and spiritual wellbeing can be achieved by a herbalist easier than other non-natural medical philosophies. A person should know what is happing behind a specific healing process so that the complexities of human nature can be well understood and fewer chances of getting side effects. As a herbalism expert, it is essential to know the basic properties of a herb/plant. It is highly essential to know the biological and spiritual aspects of a human body so that the maximum impacts of herbs can be obtained by using specific plants and herbs.

Another important aspect of herbalism practice is to use the plant as a source of deep emotional attachment so that it can be grown in full capacities with compassion and care. A herbalist should know how to grow a specific herb/plant in multiple environments and soil conditions, which can be ideal for the maximum growth of a plant. This book will cover all these necessary steps of herbalism philosophy in the easiest possible ways so that new readers and fresh herbalism students can find the fundamental essence of herbalism.

Specific terminologies related to herbalism:

Herb is a diverse word, and different people have different thoughts on it. Herbalism as "using the herb" is not a complete meaning to it.

The meanings attached to herbalism evolved in every passing century, and it has suffered a significant dynamic change also because of the reflection of the medical world from herbal to other types. Herbal medicine was the origin of all types of medicine, but the constant change of the technological world has caused many disturbances among the basis and evolution of herbal medicine. The definition of herb, according to oxford, is related to its physical nature. According to this definition, the herb is only the type of plant which doesn't have any wooden stem and which can die after flowering. The other part of the definition focuses on its uses, and the herb is a type of plant which is used in medicine, fragrance, and oils. Many botanist definitions consider the physical nature of herbs, i.e., non-woody stem and short life span.

However, the ecologists consider herbs as plants that are shorter than 12 inches. In culinary art, some herbs are edible, and others are not. In the medical world, herbs are only those plants that have curative capacities and which can be used as a source of treatment. However, this definition doesn't include other uses of herbs. Phytotherapy considers herbs as plants which have healing capacities and can treat human as a whole.

Botany has its roots form herbalism, and before its evolution, herbalism was used instead of botany as the study of plants. It shows the historical importance of neglected herbalism. Accordingly, a person who has the profession of selling the herbs and products made by herbs is called a herbalist. Most specifically, the herbalist is a person who grows, prepares, uses herbs for a variety of purposes, and treats illnesses through herbs is called herbalist.

So, from an author's point of view, herbalism can be defined as a study or practice of the relationship between plant and human. It encompasses all the physical, medical, biological, or pharmacological aspects of a herb in the betterment of humankind.

Different types of herbalism:

Herbalism is being practiced for centuries in nearly every country and area of the world. Nearly every religion, every race, and every culture has specific uses of herbs for different purposes. Medical uses of herbs are the most prominent ones. A herbalist is very important in preserving the specific botanic culture and plant preservation of a specific area. It is not just the use of herbs for medical purposes; herbalism encompasses the specific relationship between man and plant. Nearly every era of time and every area of the world has its own specific herbalist system of practice, which includes the Islamic system of herbal medicine, Indian era or herbalism, Chinese herbalism, and western herbalism. Homeopathy and therapeutic use of aroma are some examples of western herbalism.

Orthodox medicine also has its core from herbalism school of thought, which believes that any medical system which provides benefits and prevents hazards to human health can be practiced freely without any difference. However, the basic principles related to herbalism and the use of herbal medicine have shaken to its core due to cultural differences and more conflicted flow of modern western medicine. The use of herbs for health will never fade away, and recently, the modern system of medicine is again utilizing the benefits of herbal medicine for the betterment of humankind.

Herbalism versus different medical systems:

Homeopathy:

Homeopathy has a relevant historical background, and it is often misperceived as herbalism. However, homeopathy and herbalism have many fundamental differences. The misconception related to the similarity of both professions is due to the use of plants. There are many differences in therapy styles and principles related to the use of herbs in both schools. Homeopathy has also been demoralized and disrespected in regard to its use; however, this text will only differentiate the scope of both valuable professions. Like can be used to cure the like is the basic principle of homeopathy, which has its origin from the early 1800s, and it is used in nearly every country with a limited scope of practice. The primary use of herbs in homeopathy is to produce very dilute solutions to avoid side effects. Nearly 55% of homeopathic medicine uses herbs as a source of cure, and it also uses a holistic approach to treat human illnesses. Other sources of medicine are minerals and salts. The diluted solutions are introduced in the human body to drive the principle forces within the body to cope with the illnesses. The dose-potency relationship between medicine and the human body is inverse in homeopathic philosophy. According to homeopaths, if higher doses of herbs cause illness, a very diluted dose of these herbs can treat the symptoms as well (like treats like), and it is the fundamental difference among homeopaths and a herbalist.

There are so many herbs that are used by both herbalists and homeopaths, and interestingly, these herbs are used for the same illnesses in both professions. So, the misconception of similarity between both these professions is very valid. However, the underlying philosophies attached behind the user can differentiate the idea of using herbs for curing illnesses in homeopaths and herbalists.

Homeopathy is indeed a successful way of treating illnesses, and it uses herbs for sure, but the philosophies and principle related to homeopathy are not botanical in nature, and by the use of proper knowledge of both professions, a visible difference can be made by from styles of treatment and types of remedies.

Allopathy:

Interestingly, allopathic use of medicine is most common today, and the founder of homeopathic medicine used this word for the first time to differentiate homeopathy from herbalism. The modern-day practice of medicine is based on chemical salts that are made in laboratories and don't have a natural core to produce the medicine. The use of the word "allopathic" is actually not justified for modern medicine because it has its historical background with herbalism. In modern medicine, there is no to very little use of herbs in their natural forms, and compounds are prepared in laboratories. This is very different from herbalism in which plants and herbs are grown and used in their most natural forms to treat the illnesses. Modern medicine also lacks in the holistic approach and mostly uses the term "treat the cause" to ensure a healthy life. However, in herbalism, the use of human nature as a whole, i.e., mind, body, and spirit is essential to promote the complete form of wellness as described by WHO. There is a historical rivalry in both professions because it is thought that modern medicine has outraced the herbalism by using false propagandas about it. However, herbalism also lacks in solid research background as compared to modern medicine, which is a drawback of herbalism school of thought. There should be no difference among any type of treatment methodology until it is beneficial for human beings with minimum side effects.

Herbalism:

Herbalism is by far the most historical type of medical treatment strategy implemented by nearly every era of the human race and in every country of the world. Herbalism is the use of herbs for therapeutic purposes and poses a deep relationship between man and plant. It is widely practiced by every human culture, race, or religion. Herbalism is the most natural type of medical treatment in which herbs are grown and used to reduce the risks associated with herbs. A wide variety of different methods are implicated in using herbs for therapeutic purposes. Tinctures, solutions, grains, oils, and many other forms of herbs are used as a medication to treat nearly every system of the human body.

A herbalist is a person who grows, prepares, and uses herbs to treat the illnesses related to the human mind, body, and spirit. Herbalism has its basis on holistic pharma in which physical, emotional, and spiritual aspects of the human body are treated instead of just treating the cause. It is very different than homeopathy, allopathy (modern medicine), and other types of medical schools in treating human illnesses.

Evaluation of herbs for medical uses:

Herbs are used by herbalists to cure human illnesses in multiple forms and remedies. The quality control of herbs, as well as the underlying processes imposed by these herbs to cure the diseases, is highly essential to understand to avoid risks and dangers related to toxicity and overdose. Many other factors are also used to assess the quality of a herb.

Organoleptic analysis:

The use of human organs or, more specifically, the human senses to assess something is called the organoleptic analysis. Human being has five senses, i.e., smell, sight, taste, touch, and hearing. The first four senses are crucial to assess the quality of a herb. It will give a rough idea about the freshness and odor of a herb. The quality of the herb is organoleptic analysis is not sufficient until further analysis is carried out to confirm the safety issues related to herbs.

Microscopic analysis:

The use of a microscope becomes essential when the herb is assessed in its powdered form. Not every herb is fresh and safe for human use, and it can also contain some harmful pollens, fungi, algae, bacteria, and viruses. Microscopic analysis confirms the presence or absence of these microorganisms in powdered herbs.

Physical analysis:

Crude nature, melting point, shape, texture, color, and weight are some essential aspects of a herb that can be assessed by carrying out a physical analysis of herbs. It is essential because it gives a specific private label to a herb about its dosage and texture.

Chemical analysis:

Chemical analysis is essential to know about the chemistry of a herb. It is essential to carry out a chemical analysis because it will give essential ideas about the toxicity, dosage, or uses of a herb. Amino acid content, fats, carbohydrates, vitamins, minerals, alkaloids, acids, poisons, and many other critical chemical aspects of a herb can only be found by carrying out specific chemical analysis. It is by far the most important type of analysis related to quality control ad usage of a herb and can only be carried out by experts. Different types of chromatography (gas, liquid, weight) are used to know about the specific chemical nature of a herb. An herbalist must seek professional help to carry out these chemical analyses.

Biological analysis:

Another critical analysis that shows the specific biological characteristics of a herb as well as to assess the impacts of herbs on biological responses of the body. The biological analysis encompasses the specific measures to calculate the proper dosage of a herb. It can be a hit and trial method, and cadaver studies are carried out in which animals are used first to assess the specific impacts of a calculated dose of the herb in order to get the right idea about its impact on the human body. Another use of biological analysis is to measure the level of toxicity that can be occurred by overdosing the herb. It can also lead to catastrophic impacts when a dose is given above a standard dose. Toxicology is the study of toxicity related to any compound which is introduced in the human body. From a broader perspective, biological analysis is also used to check specific impacts of a herb on specific organ systems/systems in the human body so that a complete code can be formulated specifying the uses and dosage of a herb to benefit the human body.

CHAPTER 2: HISTORY OF HERBALISM AND HERBAL MEDICINE:

Traditional ways to treat human illnesses spanned hundreds and thousands of years to evolve into so-called modern medicine. Human, from its evolution, has used plants as a source of cure to human illnesses. Traditional Chinese ideology about medicine also used herbs as a fundamental source of healing, and this philosophy considers human as an evolving and dynamic nature which can self-heal if provided with the right environment. According to this theory, a dynamic balance between matter and energy is crucial to seek the complete form of health and wellbeing.

The use of the healing capacities of nature to cure illnesses and self-healing is an essential term in traditional Chinese medicine. The term is also used by herbalism and other natural schools of medical treatment. Western medicine is based on matter, and the energetic component is entirely absent in it. This system of medicine only incorporates those things which can be seen and can be calculated, and energies can only be felt and hard to calculate, a western system of modern medicine has entirely abolished its use in healing capacities. A specific code of conduct and a global communication system with uniform terminologies is an essential step in transferring and communicating on a variety of topics related to health and medicine. A complete form of health can only be achieved when all aspects of health are taken into consideration and uniformly implemented. The use of matter and energy as described in traditional Chinese medicine, as well as the holistic approach in traditional western management, lead to achieving a complete form of health in which no illness is present in the physical nature of the human body as well as human as a whole. There are multiple traditional concepts of medicine that were used by different regions, eras, and religions. Some of these ideologies have their roots extending from thousands of years. The most important historical aspects of traditional medicine that use herbs as an essential component to achieve maximum health status are Traditional Indian medicine, Traditional Chinese medicine, Traditional Egyptian medicine, Roman and Greek era of medicine, traditional Islamic medicine, and Western/American traditional medicine. This chapter of the book will, through brief light on the evolution of these traditional health systems and their use of herbal medicine to cure human illnesses.

Traditional Indian medicine:

The oldest documents available on herbal medicine have origin in India in which ayurvedic medicine was used as a base of the health system. This system is solely comprised of using herbs as a base of the health and integrity of the human body. Pandits and Swamis of Indian culture were thought to be the medical practitioners as well as the religious bodies who could cure the human illnesses of physical, emotional, or spiritual nature. Herbs were always an essential component of traditional Indian medicine. These herbs were used in multiple forms to cure a variety of diseases. Some herbs were also used for magic and spiritual purposes. Indian traditional medical system is not entirely dead and is being practiced in India, as well as it is widely known to other countries during modern times too. The lively nature of this system which makes it fit even after thousands of year is because the natural sources of treatment which can never die till the Day of Judgment.

Traditional Chinese medicine:

The first written document about herbal medicine in Chinese is almost 5000 years old. Traditional Chinese medicine is unique in the use of terminologies like ying-yang and ashi points. Traditional Chinese ideology about medicine also used herbs as a fundamental source of healing, and this philosophy considers human as an evolving and dynamic nature which can self-heal if provided with the right environment. According to this theory, a dynamic balance between matter and energy is crucial to seek the complete form of health and wellbeing. The use of the healing capacities of nature to cure illnesses and self-healing is an essential term in traditional Chinese medicine. The term is also used by herbalism and other natural schools of medical treatment. Meridians were the terms used along with ashi points in Chinese medicine according to which energy can be trapped in these points (ashi points), and constant flow of meridians (energy) is essential for the complete health of a human being. Along with acupuncture and cupping therapy, herbal use of medicine was the most critical aspect of Chinese medicine. A large variety of herbs were utilized by ancient Chinese doctors to cure the imbalances between matter and energy, which were thought of as an essential basis of illnesses in human bodies. Western modern medicine is entirely different from the ancient Chinese system of medicine because in the western system, the only focus of interest is the matter, and energies are heavily neglected in modern western medicine because it can't be seen or calculated.

Traditional Egyptian medicine:

The culture at the bank of Neil is nearly 8000 years old. Along with the spectacular pyramids of Egypt, this culture also had amazing medical backgrounds. Herbs were considered as the most important remedies to cure human illness as well as in magic. The pharaoh of Egypt used special herbs to enhance their sexual and physical powers, as well as magic, had a strong base in Egyptian culture. Herbs had a crucial part in religious ceremonies and cultural events. The proofs of herbs used in medicine, as well as other aspects, can be seen through the walls of the great pyramids.

Roman and Greek era of medicine:

In the Roman and Greek empires, medicine is thought to be evolved. The base of modern medicine rooted back in the Roman and Greek era, and Hippocrates was the most phenomenal physician of that time. The excellent writings of Hippocrates also suggest that the herbal use of medicine was the primary and most fundamental part of the ideology of healing. Herbs were used to treat wounds of soldiers, to increase sexuality and strength, and to cope up with epidemics and illnesses. It is obvious to say that the Greek and

Roman empire promoted the use of herbal medicine, but the modern medical system has disrespected this crucial base of the healing system.

Traditional Islamic medicine:

Islam is one of the most followed religions in the world, and its history is nearly 1400 years old. In the Islamic system of medicine, the word Tibb was used, and Tabib was the doctor who was eligible to practice medicine. Avicenna is known as the father of biology, who was a Muslim scientist of the same era. There are thousands of books and proofs in Islamic literature that show that the traditional Islamic system of medicine was based on herbal medicine. Herbs were used in calculated doses to treated illnesses related to human bodies. Some herbs were used for aromatherapy and perfumes as Arabic culture is rich in the use of aroma called It, which is based on herbs.

American/western traditional medicine:

The basic concept of the Chinese system of medicine has a fundamental rule of harmony and balance among matter and energy. There should be a balance in the dynamic nature of humans to achieve health in the Chinese system. The same concept is utilized by the western holistic approach of medicine in which a person should be treated as a whole rather than treating just the symptoms. A western holistic doctor works on the mind, body, and spirit of a person to achieve maximum health.

Vitalism is a term used by western medicine, which states that living organisms are not similar to nonliving things. Both contain physical aspects, but the living objects contain some nonphysical components like soul, emotions, and drives, which are vital for life.

Vitalism also states that illnesses occur when disturbances are encountered in the physical and nonphysical nature of a human being, which is very similar to the traditional Chinese system of medicine, which states that there should be a balance between matter and energy for complete health.

Just like chi, ashi points, and meridians, Hippocratic terminologies about four temperaments and energies are used in western medicine.

General medicine has an origin from Native or Latin Americans, which possess an era between the 19th and mid-20th centuries. It is the base of American herbalism because of the use of herbs and botanic substances along with other objects to cure the diseases. John Uri is thought of as the father of general medicine.

Vitality stands for the capacity of a human body to adapt a specific human illness and internal drive to cure it by using primary principle forces, which can be enhanced by the use of specific medicine. Nearly every medical personal used this philosophy.

Thomsonianism is a term used in the name of Samuel Thomson, who raised his voice against invasive treatments and advocated in favor of herbal use of medicine, which is more natural and safe. Samuel Thomson was an American. The medical system of the 19th century has its basis in the ideology of Samuel Thomson, and it is, therefore, reasonable to say that the American system of medicine was herbal medicine until modern western medicine came to the world.

Many times during the western medical history, art and science came hand in hand and collaborated to make a belief system which was driven by vital forces.

Physiomedicalist is a terminology used in western medicine for those who believed that some symptoms of illnesses have a positive impact on these vital forces, and some have negative impacts.

All these philosophies with some others which were prevailed and grown in western medicine culture were using herbs as a source of medical cure to the illnesses of human being, and there is no doubt to say that herbalism is the primary driving force in the growth of western medical culture and modern medicine. Natural remedies to treat the disease were more successful in this context, and invasive procedures were thought of as taboo. Mind, body, and spirit were used to be treated as a whole, and there was a significant shift in holistic medicine due to herbalism principles in western medicine.

It was thought that illnesses or diseases are due to an imbalance in natural equilibrium in the body, and this balance has to be maintained to treat the person and achieving maximum health. As discussed in the above context, it is clearly proven that western medicine culture has some fundamental basis, which is quite similar to Chinese traditional medicine and other sources of medicinal growth. So, it is essential to say that nature always played a pivotal role in anchoring the balance of life and death, and this equilibrium of nature is most important to maintain if complete health is required. Herbs are the most natural source of medicine, and the curative capacities of herbs are superior to artificially made substances, which can have more side effects than the benefits.

It is also vital that the body's natural capacity to cope up with illnesses is highly essential to maintain this natural equilibrium. Herbalism is believed that by providing some natural resources yielded from the herbs, the body's capability to cope with the stress related to illness can be enhanced to many folds. This is much similar to the self-heal theory of Chinese traditional medicine, which is also used by western traditional medicine experts. Form menopause to liver disorders, everything can be cured by herbs. Lignans and phytosterols are essential in providing the cooling and buffering effects on the liver and thus reduce the chances of getting cirrhosis and many other hepatic abnormalities. Isoflavones and phytosterols are essential compounds to boost the endocrinal functions of the human body. Patience is required when practicing herbalism because without patience; there will be no effect on any drug. Herbs are grown with time and in care and compassion. Similarly, it is essential to seek patience when using them for health. Time is always required to boost the inherent capabilities of a body to channel the self-healing impacts. Herbal medicine may take longer than allopathic chemical compounds to heal some illness, but the side effects associated with the right herbs are very less than synthetic and artificial compounds. This makes herbal medicine as a treatment of choice in many cases.

In relevant chapters of the book, uses of different herbs on specific illnesses and body systems will be discussed in detail.

CHAPTER 3: WHY TO CHOOSE HERBALISM OVER OTHER SCHOOL OF THOUGHTS

Herbalism is by far the most historical type of medical treatment strategy implemented by nearly every era of the human race and in every country of the world. A wide variety of different methods are implicated in using herbs for therapeutic purposes. Tinctures, solutions, grains, oils, and many other forms of herbs are used as a medication to treat nearly every system of the human body. A herbalist is a person who grows, prepares, and uses herbs to treat the illnesses related to the human mind, body, and spirit. Herbalism has its basis on holistic pharma in which physical, emotional, and spiritual aspects of the human body are treated instead of just treating the cause. It is very different than homeopathy, allopathy (modern medicine), and other types of medical schools in treating human illnesses.

It is essential to know that WHO believes that any medical system which provides benefits and prevents hazards to human health can be practiced freely without any difference. However, the basic principles related to herbalism and the use of herbal medicine have shaken to its core due to cultural differences and more conflicted flow of modern western medicine. The use of herbs for health will never fade away, and recently, the modern system of medicine is again utilizing the benefits of herbal medicine for the betterment of humankind. The high strength of herbalism expert is the integration of traditional philosophies of healing with modern day scope of practice. Medical herbalism is very simple and highly complex at the same time. It is merely that a patient can get the maximum benefit of a weed by just growing it in his/her backyard and chewing it or drinking the dissolved solution. The complexities lie in the fundamental biochemical and pharmacological aspects of a herb using as a treatment of choice.

The self-healing strategy used by a medical herbalist is to introduce a patient about a specific herb and providing him knowledge of proper uses and benefits of that specific herb. He/she makes the patient eligible to grow his/her own weed or herb and thus, provides a higher degree of autonomy to the patient. From a seed to a complete plant, a patient seeks close attachment with the growth of that plant, and thus, the benefits on the mind, body, and spirit of a patient introduced by the plant are many folds. In medical herbalism practice, a properly educated patient works in close coordination with a plant that not only cures his/her physical illnesses but also helps in experience a whole new life, from a seed to a full-grown plant.

<u>Herbalism vs. homeopathy:</u>

Herbal medicine may take longer than allopathic chemical compounds to heal some illness, but the side effects associated with the right herbs are very less than synthetic and artificial compounds. This makes herbal medicine as a treatment of choice in many cases. Homeopathy has a relevant historical background, and it is often misperceived as herbalism. However, homeopathy and herbalism have many fundamental differences. Nearly 55% of homeopathic medicine uses herbs as a source of cure, and it also uses a holistic approach to treat human illnesses.

<u>Herbalism vs. allopathy:</u>

Interestingly, allopathic use of medicine is most common today, and the founder of homeopathic medicine used this word for the first time to differentiate homeopathy from herbalism. The modern-day practice of medicine is based on chemical salts that are made in laboratories and don't have a natural core to produce the medicine. In modern medicine, there is no to very little use of herbs in their natural forms, and compounds are prepared in laboratories. This is very different from herbalism in which plants and herbs are grown and used in their most natural forms to treat the illnesses. Modern medicine also lacks in the holistic approach and mostly uses the term "treat the cause" to ensure a healthy life. However, in herbalism, the use of human nature as a whole, i.e., mind, body, and spirit is essential to promote the complete form of wellness as described by WHO.

<u>Herbalism vs. surgery:</u>

In surgery, the cuts and lacerations induced by the surgeons are enough to differentiate it from herbalism. In the historical era, surgeons used herbal medicine to treat the wound and associated illnesses. They used herbs and disinfectants during the procedure. In the modern world, surgery is widely practiced under the umbrella of allopathic medicine. No other medical classifications, including the herbalists, are allowed to practice invasive procedures. This is not a fair game, indeed, and it is a step of demoralizing the herbalism. Invasive procedures are not always practiced by a herbalist, but the level of misconceptions and lack of trust in herbalism is dangerous to this noble profession. The risk factors associated with surgery are many folds, and most of the allopathic surgical procedures are carried out in most unnatural ways, which can lead to many risks associated with surgeries. Herbal medicine, on the other hand, is the safest know type of treatment methodology incorporated to cure the illnesses associated with human bodies.

There are many other types of medical, paramedical, and alternative classifications of the medical hierarchy, but the debate will be too long for this essential text. The point to be raised in context to this discussion is the superiority of herbal medicine over other medical methods because of the very natural and holistic approach.

CHAPTER 4: DETAILS ABOUT CLASSIFICATION OF PLANTS USED IN HERBALISM

There are a wide variety of plants in this world. Many types of these plants are edible and human friendly. Some types of plants are notorious and carnivores. Some can grow in the dark while some need sunlight for photosynthesis. Some can be hazardous for human health, while others can benefit human health by curing many illnesses and diseases. Some plants have very potent disinfectant properties, which can be used against many types of deadly viruses and bacteria. A separate volume in this series is spared to discussed the antiviral and antimicrobial benefits of plants that are used in medical herbalism.

This chapter will through light on the beneficial details about the plants which are associated with human health and which are integral to essential medical herbalism practice.

Classification on the basis of different characteristics:

The classification systems relevant to the medicinal use of plants used by herbalists or other natural curers depend upon many characteristics and uses. Classification of medicinal plants leads to an easy and effective strategy to reduce the time of finding the suitable plant type(s) in context to a specific disease and illness. Classification can also be made on the basis of specific uses of plants as well as according to the area of production and alphabetical orders. The most common type of classification system includes various parameters, and all will be discussed in detail here.

In alphabetical order:

Binomial names of plants are in Latin, which can be used as a classification method, or plants can be used on the basis of their common names. It is all the game of personal choice. However, it is the purest form of classification.

On the basis of taxonomy:

Family, genus, or species are the classifications related to botanic culture. A botanist can classify the medicinal plant of the basis of taxonomy, which, by far, is the most professional type of classification system.

On the basis of morphology:

In this classification system, plants are classified on the basis of how they look and what characterizes they have in regard to their visible morphology. Organized drugs are based on those plants which have visible texture and uniformity among the family and genus. For example, plants can be classified as leafy or flowery, fruity or stem, etc. Unorganized drugs are based on plant extracts that don't have uniform morphology, for example, juice, gum, wax related to medicinal plants.

Therapeutic purposes:

The pharmacological benefits shown by medicinal plants can be used to classify them, and it is also an essential type of classification because it gives a clearer idea about the pharmacology of a plant.

Action-based classification:

in this type of therapeutic classification, plants are classified in regard to their actions, which are performed on different organs or organ systems of the body. They can have a cooling effect on the liver or soothing effects for gums. It is an important type of classification.

According to systems of the body:

This type of classification specific details about the organs is essential in regard to the effects of herbal medicine. Plants are classified on the basis of human organ and organ systems.

Classification on the basis of medical systems:

The traditional Chinese or Indian ayurvedic medicine system utilizes specific terminologies for different types of medicinal plants. This is also a valid statement for different other medical systems that incorporate plants as a source of healing. Medical system classification related to these terminologies for plants are diverse

Biochemical system of classification:

Saponins, alkaloids, and some other types of flavones are the terms that are related to the biochemical properties of medicinal plants. This classification system needs expertise because the biochemical names are not widely used among general practice. This classification system can also be very misleading because of the fact that the plants can be termed on the basics of organic sources of drugs, and many other essential components can be lost.

Biogenetic type of classification:

The genetic aspect in relation to the origin of a medicinal plant is a substantial base to classify this type of system. This is not a very widely used type of classification, but it can still be essential to show the geographic and historical benefits of a medicinal plant.

Geographical classification:

This type of classification is by far one of the simplest types of classification, and it incorporates a different type of geographical parameters to classify a plant. There are many countries in this world, and each country has multiple types of soils and habitats. Some countries have freezing weather while some others are tropical and contain more than three types of weather. This rich geographical diversity is an essential factor in classifying the plants on the basis of their origin. Some plants are concrete to the culture of a specific country. Some are even worshiped as the sources of higher benefits in some areas, while other types of medicinal plants are prevalent in nearly every area of the world.

So, to conclude this discussion, it is essential to say that there are multiple types of classification systems related to medicinal plants, and a herbalist should have a clearer idea and knowledge about all types of classifications or systems. A herbalist also has a huge responsibility to preserve the habitat in which a plant grows. Growing a plant is giving life, so it is crucial to treat a living organism with genuine compassion and care. The most prevalent benefit of being a herbalist is working in close coordination with plants. A herbalist never discriminates between specific classes of plants and treats them equally with love and care. This is a valuable exercise to make him more human-friendly as well and providing him an opportunity to seek love for all races, colors, and nationalities. Being a herbalist is indeed a blessing, and a patient who is treated by a herbalist should also know these points because these are essential to make him eligible for growing his own herbs with love and care.

CHAPTER 5: HERBS AS HEALING REMEDIES

To understand the health benefits of a plant, it is essential to the basic properties of that plant as well as necessary actions of the same plant on different organs and systems of the body. Our body is very complex, and any missing detail can lead to catastrophic effects. The dose of a herb given in specific illnesses should also be very calculated. In this text, we will discuss some fundamental details about nearly each and every plant used in herbalism as a source of herbal medicine.

Acerola

- *Malpighia glabra is the Latin name of this plant*
- This plant comes from Barbados cherry family
- It is fruity in nature.

Details:

This herb is essential because of unusual Vitamin C concentrations and flavin related compounds called flavonoids. It can also have nearly 3900mg of vitamin C, which makes it a perfect choice to boost natural immunity. A little weight of this plant can provide a very high amount of vitamin C so that hypervitaminosis can be a concern. It is also very rich in amazing and effective antioxidants as well as it can also contain a high amount of protein, minerals and salts, iron, and potassium. It also contains calcium and some trace minerals. Another benefit of using acerola as a daily diet is its antifungal actions. It can also be considered as a super fruit. Regular supplementation of this fruit can delays aging and prevention of many deadly and common diseases.

Dosage:

nearly 400-4500mg when used as an extract. In powder form, the required dose is nearly 3-9 grams.

Traditional use:

It is a traditional drink of Brazil, and it is considered as an effective remedy for intestinal issues and frequent fevers. It is also associated with its anti-inflammatory benefits, which can directly affect the liver, heart, and kidneys. It is also used to cure blood-related issues, rheumatic problems, and increased obesity.

Alpha-lipoic acid:

It is also known as S or R-lipoic acid.

Details:

It is also an essential supplement that is widely used in herbalism to cure many disorders and to prevent many diseases. Carrots, yams, and beef, as well as another type of red meat, are rich in alpha-lipoic acid. It has significant impacts on the energy supply of the body called ATP. It also has global effects on the body and can benefit nearly every organ and system of the body, including skin, liver, kidney, heart, and pancreas. It also has many antioxidant benefits, which makes it fit for everyday use. In cells of the body, alpha-lipoic acid contributes to enhancing the power of power grid units called mitochondria. It has been proved in cadaveric studies that alpha-lipoic acid is highly essential in treating age-related changes in the brain. It is a significant health supplement for patients of Parkinson's and Alzheimer's diseases.

It is a very natural type of COX-2 inhibitor, which is used as an anti-inflammatory and pain killer agent in many allopathic drugs. It is also very rich in glutathione and vitamin C. All these characteristics make it a perfect supplement of daily use.

Dosage:

40-350mg in R-lipoic acid

150-2000 mg as alpha-lipoic acid

<u>**Amla or Indian berry:**</u>

- *Phyllanthus Emblica* is the Latin name of this plant.
- Amla is an Indian plant, also known as Indian berry.
- It is used as whole fruit, oil extracted, and in powder form.

<u>Details:</u>

It is a flowery plant, as well as a fruit that is berry shaped. The important factor is the nutritious benefits provided by this fruit, which is rich in very unique and rare benefits. It is an important fruit which can be used in health promotion and anti-aging. It is also called as a super fruit. A vast scientific literature is dedicated to supporting this fruit. It contains high amounts of antioxidants, antifungal, antiviral, disinfectant, and protecting benefits. It is also essential In the reduction of cholesterol from the body and thus reduces the chances of atherosclerosis and heart attacks.

A word Rasayana is used in traditional Indian medicine, which is associated with the global benefits of amla in the human body. Amla is a natural coolant that can be a protective remedy during hot summers. It also has cooling effects on the liver and stomach.

<u>Therapeutic dosing range:</u>

When extracted, amla can be used in 70-1100mg dose.

When in powdered form, the daily dose can be 4-9 grams per day.

<u>Traditional uses:</u>

A word Rasayana is used in traditional Indian medicine, which is associated with the global benefits of amla in the human body. Amla is the natural coolant that can be a protective remedy during hot summers. It also has cooling effects on the liver and stomach.

It is a natural thirst reliever, and thus it is traditionally used in hot climates of India from ancient times. During Indian fasts, which can be forty-day long, amla is used as a protective fruit that can heal the body and protects from getting sick. It is also given to children mixed with sugar to protect them from evil eyes in traditional Indian culture.

Ashwagandha:

- *Withania somnifera* is called in Latin as well as botanically.
- It is also a plant of Indian origin that is widely used for its protective benefits.

Details:

It is a well-known root that is used to relieve pain and other symptoms of joint arthritis, gouty arthritis, stress and anxiety disorder, and sleep disturbances. It is also used to relieve symptoms of asthma and chronic cough. In pregnant females, it is used to relieve issues related to pregnancies, and it is also a natural cure for infertility. Patients with low libido drive and impotence can use this root for sexual benefits.

It is also an essential treatment for aging, and it can cure edema as well as age-related changes in the brain and skin. Its effects on TB and other pathogenic disorders, however, need to be established by medical research.

<u>*Dosage:*</u>

When used in crude quality, 3-9 gram is sufficient.

1-2 ml in fluid form

80-800mg in standard extract

<u>Astragalus</u>

Astragalus membranaceus is the Latin name of this plant. It is of Leguminosae (bean) subclass. It is a widely used plant in China, Japan, and Korea. It is basically a root in morphology

<u>*Details:*</u>

The importance of this root plant in traditional Chinese herbalism is well known. It is considered a great root to promote the self-healing capacity of the body and to maintain vital forces inside the body. Some western herbalists also used this root as the primary source of tonic, which is essential to promote natural immunity and vital capacities of the body. This root has some fantastic impacts on neural and endocrinal systems of the body. It can be a primary herbal remedy for patients with deficient immunity or those who are treated by chemotherapy and radiotherapy.

These benefits of the herb make it a herbal remedy of choice for cancer patients all over the world. It is a primary adaptive herbal remedy in oncology. Moreover, the use of astragalus is hazard-free and safe. It has a fantastic impact on bone marrow, and thus, it can easily promote immunity by producing more potent white blood cells that can be used in the war against the deadly pathogens like bacteria and viruses.

The research base of this root for cancer patients is highly relevant to establish its efficacy in the oncology department. It acts on multiple systems of cancer patients and promotes a more safe and healthy lifestyle in cancer patients. This herb is also essential in maintaining health benefits. It has a sweet taste, and it can be used as a powder in cancer patients. The pleasant taste of this herb is essential in more tolerance by cancer patients.

Many recipes associated with this herb promote the use of the herb in the form of smoothies because of its sweet taste and pleasant smell. This fluid form is more consumable for cancer patients. It also helps in improving the digestive health of cardiac patients.

dosage:

10-30 grams when used as a tea or smooth.

To make tea, roots slices can be boiled for several minutes, and this technique is derived from traditional Chinese medicine, which also widely practiced in many countries of the world.

When used as a fluid extract, 5-10 ml is sufficient.

Traditional uses:

It has traditional backgrounds for the betterment of vital forces inside a human body. It is a fantastic remedy for weakness, fevers, lack of immunity, deprived focus, aging, and, most importantly, cancer. *Huangqi* is the term which is used as a source of yellow energy, and it is associated with the beneficial use of this herb in

Chinese folk medicine. It is named as yellow energy because, in Chinese culture, yellow energy is thought to be associated with the vital forces inside a body which are essential to maintain equilibrium between health and illness. Qi or chi is used as positive energy, and it is thought that this herb is essential in achieving the positive energy in many human organs and systems, especially in the spleen. So, it can be easily understood that the reasons for using this herb in cancer patients are not from a lame theory, but actual uses of this herb against low immunity are clearly shown in the literature.

In China, this root is used as a symbol of defending the energy of the body, and in western medicine, it is synonymous with the word immunity. In traditional Chinese medicine, this root was also used for fever, cough, constipation, diarrhea, vomiting, and flu. It is thought that this herb can be a sufficient insufficient blood flow of the body, and thus, it can be used against peripheral vascular diseases, varicose veins, anemia, and many other blood disorders.

Bacopa

- *Bacopa monnieri* is the Latin name of this herb.
- It belongs to the family of figwort stem.
- Brahmi is another common name of this root.
- It consists of stems and leaves.

Details:

Hyssop water or bacopa is a widely known herb that contains stems and leaves. It has historical use in ayurvedic medicine, and it is being used for many centuries. Brahma means the universe Indian language, and thus it is called Brahmi because of its universal benefits. Brahmi is also a name if the goddess in India. As with amla, bacopa is also used as Rasayana in Indian medicine, which is used in the treatment of sleep deprivation, anxiety, fatigue, and stress as well as to promote brain health. It is also considered as an essential remedy to promote memory and focus. It causes an increase in concentration, which is essential for learning. Some literature also allows it to use for epilepsy. One of the most potent benefits of this herb is to slow down aging and prevent age-related changes in the brain and skin. It also has some cosmetic uses as well.

 In both India and Pakistan, the use of Bacopa is multipurpose, and it is thought of as a symbol of complete health and wellness. Bacopa is abundant in some steroid-related substances, which are essential precursors of sex hormones in both males and females. It has significant impacts on GABA receptors of the brain, which are essential to promote memory and decrease pain. It also has cholinergic benefits, which are essential in the promotion of concentration and to improve short term and long term memories. This is the reason. Yogis are using tea made of bacopa from hundreds of years to promote the focus and concentration during meditation. In children, regular use of bacopa is essential to promote necessary primitive reflexes as well as growth milestones. In mentally disabled children, the use of bacopa can lead to better rehabilitation responses and wellness.

Another significant benefit associated with bacopa is its anti-inflammatory and antioxidant benefits, which are highly essential to boost immunity and to minimize illnesses. The research and medical literature on bacopa herb are highly sufficient to establish its safe use in children, the old age population, adults, and fitness athletes. It has killing effects on intestinal parasites, which can cause anemia and other mesentery disorders in patients of all ages but especially children.

Therapeutic dosing range:

400-1000mg of bacopa is recommended in traditional Indian medicine. Tea rich in bacopa can vary between 20-30 ml per day, and if it is used as syrup, it can be between 30-35ml per day.

The recommended use if standard fluid extract for adults is 6-12 ml per day and 5-6 ml for children.

Traditional uses:

Bacopa has rich historical importance in Indian ayurvedic medicine as well as in traditional western medicine. It was widely used to promote attention, focus, longterm and short term memory, and brainpower in both children and adults. It was also used as an effective tonic for the heart and vascular health. In some literature, it is also shown that it was also used in lung diseases.

Bilberry

- *Vaccinium myrtillus* is the Latin name of the plant.
- It belongs to the health family botanically.
- Another name of the plant is wild blueberry.
- Both leaves and berries of the plant are used in herbal medicine. Uva ursi is the name implies to the leaves of this plant, which Is used for the treatment of UTIs (urinary tract infection).

Details:

This plant belongs to the Ericaceae family, and the common name implies to this plant is a blueberry plant. It has proven benefits for eye health, and ocular pathologies can easily be treated by its herbal use. It is essential to the aging process in the eyes and to improve night vision. Cataract and ocular degeneration can be controlled by its regular use. Eye weakness and blindness affect a considerable population in the world, and using the blueberry can prevent these issues.

Dosage:

500mg of pure extract is sufficient together with all the benefits provided by this plant. If it is used in capsular form, 1-3 capsules daily can be a smart idea.

Traditional uses:

For many centuries, blueberry is the fruit of choice in western culture to make pies and cakes. Sweet dishes have an essential part of blueberries in western culture. It also has a great medicinal history in traditional western and Chinese culture. As an artist of the western era, Hildegard has allegedly used blueberries in his mystic music as a source of menses in females. Historically, blueberries were used to treat frequent cough and fever, kidney stones, intestinal bloating, liver disorders, piles, and infections of the dermis and oral mucosa. Many American herbalists of ancient times used blueberries against diabetes. It was thought of as a potent source of insulin. The use of blueberries in ocular issues is widespread. It has proven benefits for eye health, and ocular pathologies can easily be treated by its herbal use. It is essential to delay the aging process in the eyes and to improve night vision. Cataract and ocular degeneration can be controlled by its regular use. Eye weakness and blindness affect a considerable population in the world, and using the blueberry can prevent these issues.

An essential historical debate about blueberries is the use of this plant in world war 2. It was a very famous plant among the pilots of the Air force. Jam made of blueberries was used before the night attacks to prevent night blindness. Glaucoma and diabetic eye diseases were also treated by regular uses of blueberries. In Europe, surgeons used blueberries for the quick healing of wounds. Brushing, hemorrhoids, and piles are treated in herbalism by using blueberry pastes. The use of blueberries to treat diarrhea is also a debate of great importance. The fibrous nature of this fruit is essential to relieve constipation, which is the hardening of stool, and nearly every human and of every age suffer from this disorder many times in his/her life. All these historical, as well as modern times benefits, are enough to consider blueberries as a super fruit. However, the use of blueberries in Indian traditional culture is not very common because these re tough to grow in that habitat.

Cordyceps

- *Cordyceps Sinensis* is the Latin name of this plant.
- It belongs to a family of sac fungi
- Caterpillar fungus is another widely used name of this plant.

Details:

Cordyceps is widely and prominently used in traditional Chinese culture as a tonic medicine. This herb is easy to grow as well as it can be grown on larger scales. The significant benefits associated with this plant are optimizing health status. It is also used to cure lungs and renal disorders. It is also an essential herb to be used by athletes. It is essential to enhance the strength and recovery of athletes. It is a fantastic herb to lower the serum creatinine levels, which is essential for the proper functioning of kidneys. It has incredible effects on achieving health for the lungs and respiratory system. Historical use of this herb to treat pneumonia, functional lung diseases, and COPD, as well as asthma, is well established and widely practiced. It is also essential to boost endocrine health.

Dosage:

The daily recommended dose of herbal extract is 1-3 grams while is maintaining the blood concentration of herb. 3-6 grams/day is essential when used by athletes or otherwise healthy individuals for therapeutic purposes.

Traditional uses:

This herb is used for centuries in traditional Chinese medicine to relieve lungs related disorders. It is considered as a potent remedy for asthma and expectoration. It is a natural cough suppressant and necessary to relieve issues related to the overproduction of mucus and saliva. Li Chih Shen is a legendry Chinese herbalist who used this herb for lung health and to cure respiratory disorders. He used this herb in his documents to restore the balance of yin and yang among the body, which is a strong base of traditional Chinese medicine. The use of the herb for kidneys, bone marrow, and hemorrhages is well established in traditional Chinese medicine. Yang, which is essential to maintain the stress, illnesses, and disorders in the body, can be maintained by using soups mixed with some mushrooms to boost bone marrow production as described in traditional Chinese medicine.

Devil's Club

- *Oplopanax horridus* is the Latin word of this herb.
- This plant belongs to the ginseng family, and botanically, it is considered in the Araliaceae family. Another name implied to this plant is Devil's stick or Devil's walking cane. Its roots leave as well as stem are used for herbal medicinal purposes in herbalism.

- It should not be confused with the devil's claw, which is a plant grown in hot deserts.

Details:

This plant is widely produced in the northwest of America. It also contains many attributes of the ginseng family, which is essential to treat diabetes. It helps in curing the insulin resistance. It also helps in lowering the increased cholesterol levels in the blood. The most significant benefit of this herb is its use in weight loss and weight management coach, who knows its herbal impact can help his/her client to reduce some extra pounds in a natural and effective manner. This plant is really a blessing for diabetic patients because it helps in increasing the blood insulin levels and reducing the blood glucose spike after meals, which can be dangerous for pre-diabetics and full-blown diabetic patients. Its anti-inflammatory and antioxidant nature helps in recovery if cancer patients because it helps in reducing the weight and extra fat in cancer patients, which is caused due to stress. Cancer patients also possess poor insulin tolerance, and thus, it helps in this regard as well.

Dosage:

When it is used in fluid form. 2-5 ml consumption of this syrup for 2-3 times a day can be a smart idea.

Traditional uses:

It is a much-used herb in Alaska and Great Britain. It was also widely used in the folk medicine of Columbia. The most prominent benefits of using this herb are to use it against joint and gouty arthritis, common fever and cough, and against diabetes. The use of this plant against diabetes is highly prominent. Natives of Alaska were found to use a herbal drink of this plant to cure cancer. They also used it for weight reduction and lowering extra pounds from the body. The use of this plant in Alaskan natives for constipation, diarrhea, stomach and skin ulcers as well as gallstones are many folds. In some traditional and folk medicine, this herb was used to increase sexuality and libido among men, and it was also used to increase menstruation in females. It was also used to restore the proper menstruation cycle after birth. The stem, leaves, and branches of this herb were used to treat the focus, attentional and mental health among society.

Elderberry

- *Sambucus nigra* is the Latin name of this plant.
- It belongs to the moschatel family, which was previously known as Caprifoliaceae.
- Other names of this plant are American elder or common elder.
- Both barriers and leaves, as well as flowers of this plant, are used for medicinal purposes
- It has potent diuretic impacts.

Details:

Elderberry is native to American habitat; most precisely, it is grown in northwest America. It has a value of great importance in traditional western medicine. Teas made from the leaves and flowers of this herb are essential in diaphoretic purposes. This herb is highly essential in treating common flu and colds. Many tonic formulas are also used from this herb. A significant benefit of this herb is its higher concentration of flavonoids. It is a potent immunity booster and essential in preventing immune stress response. It is also used to alleviate the symptoms of common colds and runny nose. It is also very beneficial in treating fever and muscle soreness. It is used to protect children from common colds and flues in hard winters.

Dosage:

2-5 ml two times a day when used as a fluid extract.

With 5 percent flavonoids in total concentration, standard extract can be used in 400-1800mg daily.

Tea of this plant can also be used, and it is easier to make. 2-5 cups per day can be easily consumed. Tea can be made from mixing the flowers and leaves of the plant.

Traditional uses:

It was used as a source of food in red Indians for centuries. Most of the use from this herb was in dried form. Wines were made from the plant as well. This plant was a source or excellent remedy in hot summers where a drink of choice which contained a perfect amount of this plant. In traditional medicine, leaves of this plant were used for pain-relieving purposes, and they were considered as a fantastic source of boosting healing mechanisms of the body so that it was safe to apply on wounds. Native Americans were fond of using this planta s a source to relieve frequent cough, dermal disorders, and disinfection purposes.

The old flowers of this plant were used as a source of diaphoretic relief of the body. It was actually the bark of this herb, which was a source of energy and power by the Africans. The paste made from this plant was also used to treat syphilis and rheumatic arthritis. There are some literary proves as well about its uses against epilepsy.

Eleuthero

- *Eleutherococcus senticosus* is the Latin name of this plant.
- It belongs to the ginseng family, and the common name implied to this plant is Siberian ginseng.
- Its roots and aerial components are used for herbal medicinal purposes, but the research background about the root of this plant is more well-researched. It also has an Asian variant called the Asian ginseng, which is actually not ginseng in pure form.

Details:

The most researched and well-adopted plant among the herbalism all around the world is Eleuthero. It is sufficient to show the importance of this plant. There is Russian eleuthero as well, which is the base of traditional Russain herbalism. This plant is excellent for every age population. It can be used by children, the young population as well as the older population without any risks of getting side effects when used in the proper doses. This plant is widely produced in China and

Russia, and the production of this plant is not just limited to the gardens only. It can also be produced in great masses for larger populations.

It was first introduced in America during the lates 1000s, and it is also an allowed name in FDA.

Dosage:

Russian extract can be used in 4-10ml concentration daily, and when used in dried or powdered form, which made from its root, 500-900mg per day is a perfect bet to make.

Traditional uses:

The use of roots from these plants was used at least 2000 years ago. The most beneficial uses of this plant were prevention and treatment of lungs and respiratory disorders, frequent colds, and flu, as well as ensuring vital forces and energies among the body. Siberian people used this plant to ensure the peak sexual performances and decreased infections related to the STDs. It is an approved herb that can be used to treat many illnesses by the Russian ministry of health. It is used as an excellent anti-inflammatory remedy because of its significant antioxidant benefits.

Epimedium:

- *Epimedium grandiflorum* is the Latin name of the plant.
- Berberidaceae or barberry is the botanic family of this plant.
- Other names associated with this plant are horny goat weed and yin yang Huo in Chinese. This species of plants have

significant medicinal benefits over thousand of other herbs used in medical herbalism.

- It is primarily a leafy plant in morphology.

Details:

The other name of plant epimedium is horny goat weed. As the name implies, this herb has potential uses to increase the sexual capacities in humans. It is a widely used herb in the United States of America. In traditional Chinese medicine, this herb was widely associated with sexuality, and it was potentially used as sexual enhancers as well as a potent remedy to treat erectile dysfunction. An exciting tale associated with this plant is about a herder who got goats. He noticed someday during herding that some of his goats turned horny sexually after eating some sort of plant. That is why it is called horny goat weed.

Apart from sexual promotion, horny goat weed also has a lot of other health benefits as well. The most beneficial effects of this plant are delaying the aging process among men and women. Endocrinology is the term used to access the endocrine system of the body. Epimedium is highly effective in delaying the aging process by impacting the hormonal systems of a human and increasing his vital capacities. Icariin is a compound that is widely found in this plant, and it has a number of different therapeutic benefits that are essential to promote health in human beings.

Yang is associated with health promotion inside the human body. It is a kidney yang disease that means it is highly effective in promoting the maximum functioning of the renal system of humans. It is also used as a combination with a variety of different other drugs to treat some prevalent illnesses as well as advanced diseases of human nature, which can be pathogenic and transmissible.

Dosing:

When used as a tea, 1-2 cups daily containing a 3-14grams concentration of this herb is sufficient to get the desired benefits.

A fluid extract is sufficient in 2-4 ml concentration.

When used in powder form, 80-480gram of the herb in extracted form is sufficient.

Traditional uses:

A 101 bc old document is a guide to Chinese traditional medicine. The name of that medicine is unknown, but in that document, this herb was called as a herb of divinity or Divine herb of Plowman. The writer was a yang supporter. He showed that the use of this herb was very effective in promoting renal and hepatic health, and bone health with muscular power was significant when this herb was used. In Chinese traditional medicine, this herb was called yin yang Huo, and the name implies that it was the herb to arouse the goats sexually. A Chinese writer named Shannon Benojing wrote an incredible book on herbal remedies that showed the use of this herb to treat penetration related issues and to relieve pain in the penis. It was also used to increase the urinary urge as well as to increase the body's qi (chi), which is the vital force of life.

Horny goat weed is very superior to treat lung diseases like acute asthmatic attacks, chronic asthma, COPD, atelectasis as well as it was considered as a superior remedy to treat atherosclerosis, obesity, hyperlipidemia and increased levels of testosterone. It was also considered an excellent remedy to treat stroke attacks in traditional Chinese medicine. In traditional Chinese medicine, this herb was considered as the primary source to improve yan yang balance among the body and to provide a healthy qi in the body, which is the vital force of life, and this term is significant when it comes to traditional Chinese medicine.

Eurycoma

- *Eurycoma longifolia* Jac is the Latin name of this plant.
- It belongs to the tree of heaven family, also called Simaroubaceae botanically.
- It is also called Malaysian ginseng and belongs to the ginseng family of herbs. In Malaya, it is called Tongkat Ali.
- This plant consists of all significant components botanically, and it contains roots and stems, flowers, and fruits, as well as a hard bark.
- It is a heightened herb in herbalism.

Details:

Eurycoma has a history that dates back to thousands of years. It is one of the most historical plants in Malaya history. However, it is also used in modern Malaya medicine due to its fantastic health benefits. Antipyretic benefits of this herb make it highly beneficial in treating frequent fevers and colds. Antimalarial benefits of Eurycoma are essential to me, is the first-class treatment of malaria, which is caused by a mosquito. Antiulcer benefits make it a perfect choice to treat stomach ulcers because of its buffering benefits. Cytotoxic benefits of these herbs are also making headlines from a couple of years, and trials are being conducted to establish its benefits in the oncology department. It is also widely used to increased sexuality in some areas of the world. Roots of this plant are known to have agents that are important against fever and fatigue. It is also an essential remedy against blood pressure related issues. In some clinical studies, it is shown that this drug is essential to increase testosterone levels in men. The health benefits of this herb are very potent and science-backed. It is a well-researched herb that is used in many areas of the world. Trials are continuously developing to ensure its effectiveness against many illnesses. The anticancer benefits of this herb are essential and can be a significant breakthrough in the world of herbalism.

Dosage:

200-1000mg of a standardized extract of this herb can be a great source of unlocking significant health benefits.

Traditional uses:

Tongkat Ali is the name of this plant in Malaya. It is the most well-known herb in the country. The most profound benefit of this herb is associated with male fertility and sexual power. A decoction made by soaking the root in water Is used to increase the male sexual capacities in Malaysia. Another use of this herb in Malaysia is in the form of a soaked tea, which is essential to treat fever and gastric ulcers. It is also instrumental in killing the parasites and worms present in the abdomen. A painkiller balm is made from the root to treat the backache, vertebral disc issues, muscle spasm, and herniation. Another benefit of using this herb is to protect or treat the symptoms of syphilis and mouth ulcers. Sumatra and some other areas of Malaysia are known to use this herb as an effective antipyretic and anti-inflammatory tonic. In Sabah, a district of Malaysia, people use its bark to make a decoction to relieve pain associated with the external wounds and injuries. In Riau, its root or stem is used to treat the symptoms of malaria and some other pathologies. People of Sumatra used this herb to protect the community against the fatal attacks of smallpox and other infections. In Vietnam, people are using this herb, especially the flowers and fruits of herb, to treat issues related to intestinal issues and illnesses. Malaria. In Sumatra, Eurycoma is used to protect people from smallpox.

Ginger:

- *Zingiber officinale* is the Latin name of this herb.
- It belongs to Zingiberaceae family botanically
- The most used part of this plant in the world is its root.

Details:

It is a well-known root which is used widely in every corner and every country in the world. It is used because of its millions of benefits which need no special consideration. Research background about this herb is highly sufficient to prove its benefits in the area of healthcare and medicine.

It is a Universal herbal agent. It is known as a cooking spice in most areas of the world. Moreover, its herbal uses in medicine and healthcare are not hidden, and it is one of the most used herbal medicine agents around the globe.

It is a world's well-known herbal spice and most favorite remedy to treat infections and inflammations. Many homemakers and mothers from the historical point of view used this herb to treat the most common illnesses of daily households. The most significant benefits associated with this herb are fever, pain associated with burns and injuries, and flu. It is also widely used for common colds and Asian flu. One of the most important benefits of ginger is on the mesentery. The human intestine is a loopy structure, and it is subjected to many illnesses due to food and infections. Bowel gas affects nearly every human being on earth, and every age is prone to this illness. Human bowel gases can cause abdominal distention and stress. Ginger is a historically proven remedy for gaseous issues. It is essential to maintain the primary media of intestine so that fewer infections can affect it, and it is also essential to increase the abdominal sufficiency related to the digestion and excretion of food.

Another significant benefit of ginger is its effects on respiration and common colds. Mostly in children, frequent colds and flu affect health due to common influenza viruses which involve millions of human beings around the globe every year. Ginger is essential to shield against these common influenza infections. It is also essential in clearing the breathing tracts from mouth to lungs, and thus it helps in preventing the symptoms of asthma and choking. It also helps in clearing the mucous from respiratory tracts. Another benefit of ginger is removing the foul odor of breathing. It prevents, treats, or shortens the symptoms of respiratory illnesses.

Another benefit of ginger is on indigestion and proper production of gastric juice. Gastric juice is essential to digest the food, and it helps in softening the food, which will then pass to the small and large intestines. Ginger helps in producing stomach acids in sufficient quantities to help indigestion. Gastric juice, when overproduced, can cause much sore breaths, stomachaches, and irritation. It is essential to regulate the proper concentrations of stomach acid to avoid any disturbances. Ginger is an extraordinary remedy to reduce the overproduction of gastric acid as well as increasing the underproduced amounts of gastric acid to improve the digestion issues.

The human intestine is loopy structures and extensive tracts to digest and finally excrete the food. Infection-related to the intestine can cause symptoms of diarrhea and constipation, as well as bloating and abdominal pains. Ginger helps in regulating the media of intestine, and thus it helps in improving intestinal health and helps in preventing the symptoms of diarrhea and constipation. Interestingly ginger also helps in reducing the inflammation of the intestine, which is associated with irritable bowel syndrome and many other inflammatory diseases of the abdomen.

It is a potent antioxidant herb that is essential in regulating the anti-inflammatory pathways of the body. Ginger helps in reducing the free oxygen radicals and highly reactive oxygen species, which can cause issues related to cell injury and cytotoxicity. It helps in detoxification of skin to make it more glowing and beautiful. It helps in reducing the redness and inflammation in eyes so that it makes them brighter and shiny as well. Ginger also helps in regulating the hormones of the body. So it is an important herb that is used in traditional Chinese medicine, Indian ayurvedic medicine as well as modern western medicine to treat the symptoms of impotence and low libido drive. It is a primary male aphrodisiac agent who is also associated with increase blood levels of testosterone as well as increased healthy sperms in semen.

Another essential benefit of ginger is the inhibition of thromboxane, which is essential in gathering and clotting from platelets. Thus inhibition of platelet is essential to reduce the inflammation in the body. This characteristic makes ginger a vital herb to reduce the signs of fever and common colds. Unlike other herbs already discussed in this chapter, ginger is a potent stimulating agent fr diaphoresis. This benefit makes it an excellent remedy to improve the blood flow in peripheral vessels as well as reducing the chances of blood clotting and deep venous thrombosis, which is a common problem in patients who are overweight and bedridden. It is also essential in regulating the heartrates in the body. It is a potent thermogenic herb that increases the temperature of the body and thus increases the overall metabolism of the body as well. It is an important herb to decrease the cholesterol levels from blood because of its lipolytic actions and a strong affinity with fats, which helps to excrete them from the body. It helps in increasing the saliva and production of bile from the gall bladder to increase the digestion of fats from the body and the reduction of free fatty acids from the blood. It is also an essential herb to prevent vomiting and morning sickness in pregnant females and chronically ill patients. It is an important herb to reduce the signs of osteoarthritis, rheumatoid arthritis, and gouty arthritis because of its benefits against the inflammatory mediators of the body.

The therapeutic benefits of ginger are millions, and a complete text can be dedicated to considering the details of these benefits. However, this book is a short guide for beginners abut herbalism, and all these mind-blowing benefits cannot be covered here in detail. From a herbalist point of view, ginger can be considered as the most crucial herb of the history because its use is from millions of years as well as, nearly every civilization has used this herb to gather some astounding benefits from it. Details will be covered in traditional use sections.

To conclude the benefits of ginger, it is essential to say that t can be used in every type of illness and pathology with fear of side effects or adverse reactions to the body because it is one of the most human-friendly types of herb ever known historically.

Dosing:

1-2 grams of a dried form of this herb two to three times per day is an effective strategy to unlock millions of benefits associated with this herb.

When used in the form of fluid extract, the same 1-2ml of fluid is sufficient to help reduce many illnesses when used three times daily.

When used in powdered form, 100 to 400 mg of powder twice or thrice daily can be an essential bet to make.

Some herbalists also use the super extract of this herb in 40 to 80mg concentration two to three times per day to achieve maximum benefits.

Traditional uses:

It is known that ginger was used for more than 2000 years in traditional Chinese medicine to treat nausea and vomiting related symptoms. It was also used in Chinese medicine to cure bleeding diseases because of platelet dysfunctions in the body as well in the treatment of rheumatic and gouty arthritis. Another use of ginger in traditional Chinese medicine was to treat the symptoms of snakebite and other venomous stinks. It was also a very potent herb used in the treatment of pain in gums and teeth. Stomach and intestine related issues were also treated by using this herb in traditional Chinese medicine. It is also used as an excellent remedy to treat intestinal gases and abdominal distentions. Ginger was considered as a shield against hard winters because it was an extraordinary remedy to treat the symptoms of frostbite due to its thermogenic properties. These thermogenic properties of this herb were also fundamental to treat the symptoms of cold extremities, weak and bounding pulse, cough, and fever as well as flu. Traditional Chinese medicine also used this herb in summers and damp weather.

In India, Ayurveda used this herb to prevent cardiac arrest due to blood clotting and to fight against the symptoms of atherosclerosis in the arteries of the heart. In Malaysia and other Asian countries, soups rich in ginger were given to the new mothers after delivering their babies to increase sweating and perforations so that impurities can be excreted from the body after birth. In Arabic and traditional Muslim medicine, ginger was used to increase the maleness and testosterone. In traditional African medicine, ginger is used to treat the symptoms as a mosquito repellent herb. Western traditional herbalism used this herb in the form of infusion to treat congestion and pain associated with the female menstrual cycle. Ginger has the potency to decrease pain and abdominal cramps in menstruating females. Ginger was used In nearly every culture, and it was used for nearly every type of illness of humankind due to its great health benefits. In some herbalism cultures, ginger was also used as a flavoring and fragrant agent to build different types of scents and perfumes with hundreds of therapeutic benefits. In short, ginger is a complete type of super herb in human history.

Ginseng

- Other names of this plant family are Korean and American ginseng.

- It belongs to the Araliaceae plant family.
- It is also known as Ren Shen (in traditional Chinese medicine which means human root)
- The most used part of this plant is its root.

<u>*Details:*</u>

Ginseng is a well known traditional medicine of Asia and the specific region. It is used to treat many illnesses from at least five thousand years. It has a robust research background in both traditional and modern herbalism. Nearly four hundred papers are published in favor of ginseng. Korean ginseng has the Latin name of *Panax ginseng,* and *Panax quinquefolius* is the Latin name of American ginseng. It has a distinguished title of 'LORD" of herbs in herbalism, and ginseng is a Chinese word which means man essence. In traditional Chinese medicine, the ginseng family of herbs was an essential remedy to treat and support five vital organs and organ systems (cardiac, respiratory, hepatic, renal, and spleen). It was also used to treat the balance between yin and yang. It was associated with the long life of men and women. Dr. Shiu Ying Hu is a well known Chinese herbalist who considers ginseng as an essential root of vital forces prevailing in the earth. He also considers this herb as a physical form of energy.

An American family of ginseng is sweet in taste, and it is warm in nature. It is less aggressive and stimulating as compared to Asian or Korean ginseng. In traditional Chinese medicine, yin and yang are two different personalities used for humans. It is a potent herb to be used by the young population, both male and female, from type A (yang type) personalities. American ginseng is superior to Korean and Asian ginseng because of less stimulating, having warm nature and nourishing; it is also a superior remedy to reduce symptoms of stress and fatigue. An essential benefit of American ginseng is its use against pneumonia and other lung disorders. When used regularly, it can treat and cure the symptoms of anxiety and depression. It is an extraordinary remedy to treat autoimmune disorders. A person with a known history of fatigue and tiredness can also be anemic because blood deficiency can cause these symptoms. The use of American ginseng can relieve these symptoms with overstimulation, which is the side effect of Asian and Korean ginseng. It is also a thing of standard practice that many herbalists use the combination if these American and Asian ginseng to achieve the maximum benefits of sensing family.10-20% a mixture of all types of ginseng can be the best bet to make in this regard. When ginseng is used carefully, they can also care about conditions related to insomnia. Ginseng's family of plants is very diverse in nature, with thousands of subtypes. These multiple variants of ginseng can be an issue of interest. Panax ginseng is hard to find in Russia, and thus Russian herbalist doesn't use it much frequently apart from is benefits. Some common side effects related to Russian ginseng are hyperirritability of mood and nervousness, which can be countered by diluting the source and supply of ginseng. There are around twenty-five different types of ginseng subtypes which are famous when it comes to health and wellness benefits. Out of these twenty-five ginsengs, eleven subtypes contain ginsenosides, which is a very active compound, and it is related to the health and wellness benefits. It has a variety of different benefits to treat many illnesses and diseases of human beings.

<u>*Dosing:*</u>

When used as a crude herb, ginseng can be used in two to five grams concentrations two times a day.

Fluid extract of this herb can be used 1-2 ml concentration nearly two to three times per day.

The powdered extract can be used in 100-400 mg of daily dose utilized to treat many illnesses.

Raw ginsenoside extract can be used three times a day

Green tea:

- *Camellia sinensis* is the Latin name of this herb
- It belongs to the family of Tea, also called Theaceae.
- Leaves of this plant are used for medicinal purposes.

<u>*Details:*</u>

Tea is well known and probably the most consumed beverage in the world. The use of this herb for medicinal purposes is well known and has a strong research background. Black tea requires the essential and partial fermentation process of the tea leaves. However, green tea doesn't require these kinds of fermentation and can be produced through the process of steaming the leaves. This process reduces the oxidation capacities of enzymes present in tea leaves, and the preservation of polyphenol is achieved through this process. It is interesting to know that Polyphenols belong to a family of flavonoids which are present 30-40 percent of the total weight in dried green tea leaves. Camellia sinensis is a known name of dried and unfermented green tea leaves. It has a property to reduce bacterial and viral activities in the body. It is also essential in lowering down the increased concentration of lipids in the blood. The potency of green tea to lower down the blood cholesterol level is excellent, and thus it is a beverage of choice to reduce some extra pounds from the body. It is a potent anti-lipidemic agent. Its antioxidant benefits make it a perfect choice to detoxify the liver, kidneys, intestine, stomach, and skin. Its detoxifying and lipid-lowering benefits make it a perfect choice as a natural healer. The scientific base behind green tea is solid, and it is used in traditional as well as modern medicine as a natural source to treat many common illnesses of the human body. It is a super herb in holism, and the benefits of this herb are beyond the capacity of this essential book on holism.

Dosage:

When used in crude form, 2 to 12 grams of green tea is sufficient to unlock thousands of benefits.

1-6 cups of green tea can be consumed daily without any fear of side effects.

When used as a standard extract, 200-1800 mg of green tea can do wonders for the body.

Traditional uses:

The ancient name of green tea is Camellia. It is a well-known herb in Asia for thousands of years. Camellia sinensis is a particular type of tea plant which is used to treat the symptoms of many common illnesses in traditional Chinese medicine for centuries. The oldest use of this plant in traditional Chinese medicine is present from about 500 BC. This date is already written in an ancient Chinese medicine journal; however, the real date of its use can be very long ago. A legend related to traditional Chinese medicine throws light on the discovery of green tea. The green tea plant was first discovered by a Chinese warrior named Shennong, who was nearly 5000years ago. In this regard, Chinese and Japanese royal elites enjoy a traditional ceremony called tea ceremony in memory of legendry discovery. It is essential to say that during the sixteenth century, green tea was introduced in England by the international traders who traveled across Asia and the Pacific region. It was so unique in those times that the green tea was used to be store in silver boxes of elite class homes.

Oat seed:

Avena sativa is the Latin name of this herb.

It belongs to the grass family of plants

Poaceae is the botanic name of this plant family

White seeds that are still immature are used in medicinal herbal purposes.

nervine tonic is another name of oat seed because of its significant impacts on mental health. This is a great plant that is used to treat symptoms of fatigue and stress related to the brain's health. Another benefit of this plant is to use it against many addictions, which are due to the brain's adaptability to this addictive against such as nicotine and cannabis. The withdrawal symptoms of these plants can be so intense that agitated and aggressive moods can prevail. It is a fantastic remedy to treat the symptoms of addiction. Stress is an essential factor that is associated with the brain's stress, and fatigue, and the use of oat seed an effectively treats these symptoms. This plant has fantastic benefits of restoring the body's vital energy, which also plays an essential role in preventing stress and mood disturbances.

Avena sativa is the generic name of oat seed, which is used to nourish and improve the human nervous systems. Anxiety, impaired sleep, and decreased sexual performance, which are the secondary impacts of stress, can also be treated directly by using oat seeds regularly. This plant has superior benefits over many other herbs because of having an abundant supply of vitamins and minerals in it, which are highly crucial for the proper performance of the nervous system.

Adrenal stress can also be treated by using oat seeds in these two types of formulations.

<u>*Dosing:*</u>

2-8 ml daily use of oat seed fluid extract is highly essential to unlock versatile benefits. When used in powdered form, 200-400ml of dry weight can yield thousands of benefits.

<u>*Traditional uses:*</u>

Avena sativa, also known as oat seed, is a highly crucial antispasmodic agent which is used to treat various nervous and intestinal symptoms. The traditional use of this plant is highly essential in regard to the brain's health and against anxiety and depression. It is an emotional booster and, when combined with other neurotropic agents, can provide an extremely stimulant base for mental health—different combinations of this herb along with other adaptogens utilized in herbalism.

CHAPTER 6: RECIPES FOR EVERYDAY HEALTH

In previous chapters, it is clearly described that there is a number of different methods to use herbs as a source of health and wellness. Many different herbs used in medical herbalism are also considered in detail to unlock many benefits of these herbs. It is a beginner text on medical herbalism, and only the required and most essential herbs were discussed in detail. In this chapter, some essential ways to prepare herbal medicine will be described as well as their roots of administration will also be clearly mentioned.

Combining herbs or utilizing them alone is a pure art that requires scientific knowledge and passion for humanity. An herbalist is known to deliver these benefits. Herbs can be used for symptomatic relief as well as they can also use to restore the natural balance in the whole body. The human body is unique in self-healing capacities, and these herbs can be used to promote this function of the body. However, the mastery to make useful herbs in most useable for comes with experience and trials. Sustainability and better knowledge are the most critical factors in success from herbalism. It is essential to choose the right herb and the right technique or recipe to form a right herbal medicine for a specific disease. A practical approach in this context is more beneficial rather than just theoretically learning the procedure. In this chapter, we will discuss the ways to provide this technique suitable for every possible situation or health crisis. These techniques are easy to master and comfortable to use when performed correctly and accurately according to the instructions. Some important points related to the quality of herbs, dosing, and measurement of medicine, as well as the identification of a specific herbal medicine for a specific illness, will also be described in detail. Some basic instructions of making teas and decoctions will be included in specific details along with its uses. The use of poultices, cloth application (washcloth), and heat application are also important to describe here. The use of essential oils from these herbs, as well as homemade recipes for specific oil infusions, will also be discussed. An essential technique of making herbal medicine is to use them as a tincture, and it will be covered in detail here. Then in the next chapter, a specific grouping of herbal medicine according to their uses will be discussed in detail.

Quality control and assessment of herbs:

It is a great practice to grow herbs on our own without sticking to commercial products because these home=grown herbs are more organic and safe in nature. By this process, the quality and preparation of herbs are not hidden from herbalist's eye, who grows them by his/her own hands. It is also essential to know that not every herb is capable of growing in the backyard, and many of them need a specific climate to grow. There is a clear indication to grow a specific type of herb, and it is called growing needs. A herbalist must also be capable of growing herbs in context to treat the whole mind, body, and spirit rather than ticking to specific symptoms. Planting herbs on the basis of wholesome is more accessible and more available as compared to sticking on precise details of growing herb, e.g., grown herbs for dentistry, etc.

A full-fledged garden of acres is not essential to be a herbalist. A small pot based backyard, window box, or a sitting area can be turned into an amazing botanical garden to grow amazing herbs. A self-grown botanical garden can have short sized herbs without stem or can also contain large bark containing plants. It all depends upon the specific needs of a herbalist and area available. When purchasing already grown plants form commercial nurseries, it is essential to know the specific genus and family of the plant as well as its natural health. A herbalist can distinguish between different genus and species from the same family of plants. Wildcrafting is a term that is very specific with collecting herbs from forests and wildlife rather than collecting them from nurseries. Important factors to note while working on herbs are:

1. Find a specific type of herbs.

2. Never grow herbs on contaminated areas and walkthroughs because a contaminated land can disturb the health benefits assured by medical herbs.

3. Specific herbs should be grown n in most suitable seasons only to avoid disturbances. Some species require special arrangements even when a suitable environment comes. However, some herbs are more invasive and growing in nature, for example, barriers.

4. Herbs can be purchased from commercial nurseries and shops in dried or fresh forms.

5. The integrity of herbs and their overall health must be kept in mind while purchasing the herbs from commercial sources.

6. Age of plant must also be kept in mind because, in medical herbalism, different ages of the plant have different potencies.

7. Herbs can be assessed by just looking at the color and integrity. Differences in colors and sizes can be present between the groups belonging from the same botanical families of plants.

8. More differences can be made on the aromatic nature of herbs.

9. Herbs can be very fresh or very dried, and aroma can be varied according to the type of herbs.

10. The taste of a herb is also significant while assessing the quality of the herb. A herb can be lovely too very bitter in nature. The specific quality of herbal medicine also matters to its taste. It is a common practice that herbs, which are sweeter in nature, are more consumable as compared to herbal medicines, which are sore or bitter in taste. These factors are important while assessing the compliance of patients.

11. Starting a process of herbal medicine continues from an idea to medicine in a jar, and each and every step from sowing the seed to extracting the medicine is crucial to unlocking maximum benefits provided from specific herbs.

Guidelines about dosing:

Dosing of specific herbal medicine depends upon various factors. Dose for infants is different from children. Dose for adults is different than old age population. The dose of some concentrated medicine is different than a diluted one. Dosing can also be different from a practitioner's perspective. Dosing can be made from using common observational sense as well as it can also be guided through different research trials. Infants, for example, are not the right candidate for herbal tea (twice daily); however, a 1-3 tablespoon dose can be a safe bet to make for an infant. Tinctures can vary from 5-10 drops daily for infants. Adults require much larger doses.

Acute conditions may require multiple doses per day as compared to chronic doses, which require fewer doses for a prolonged time. Herbal medicine incorporates dosage according to the individual needs of a person rather than just treating symptoms with predetermined dosing strategies. It is not essential that only the specific pattern of dosing can be used, and it can vary according to personal needs and interests, which is not practice when it comes to western allopathic medicine. Side effects of herbal medicine are also possible, which can vary from allergies to full-blown diarrhea and vomiting, so there should be a careful assessment prior, during, and after a herbal medicine treatment. Some herbalist uses a strategy of adaptation in which medicine is incorporated in much smaller doses, and dose can be enhanced periodically according to careful assessments. It is an important strategy to avoid complications related to overdosing.

Recipies and ways of preparation for herbal medicine:

Herbal medicine can be made at home in the form of teas, tinctures, washcloths, and oils. Some forms also use external ways of application, for example, baths.

Now, we will discuss a different way of herbal medicine preparation and administration at home:

Teas:

Tea is well known and probably the most consumed beverage in the world. The use of this herb for medicinal purposes is well known and has a strong research background. Black tea requires the essential and partial fermentation process of the tea leaves. However, green tea doesn't require these kinds of fermentation and can be produced through the process of steaming the leaves. This process reduces the oxidation capacities of enzymes present in tea leaves, and the preservation of polyphenol is achieved through this process. It is interesting to know that Polyphenols belong to a family of flavonoids which are present 30-40 percent of the total weight in dried green tea leaves. Camellia sinensis is a known name of dried and unfermented green tea leaves. It has a property to reduce bacterial and viral activities in the body. It is also essential in lowering down the increased concentration of lipids in the blood. The potency of green tea to lower down the blood cholesterol level is excellent, and thus it is a beverage of choice to reduce some extra pounds from the body. It is a potent anti-lipidemic agent. Its antioxidant benefits make it a perfect choice to detoxify the liver, kidneys, intestine, stomach, and skin. Its detoxifying and lipid-lowering benefits make it a perfect choice as a natural healer. The scientific base behind green tea is solid, and it is used in traditional as well as modern medicine as a natural source to treat many common illnesses of the human body. It is a super herb in holism, and the benefits of this herb are beyond the capacity of this essential book on holism.

Dosing of tea depends upon different factors and situations. When used in acute disorders and illnesses, the current complaint guides the dosage. Acute conditions may require multiple doses per day as compared to chronic doses, which require fewer doses for a prolonged time. Herbal medicine incorporates dosage according to the individual needs of a person rather than just treating symptoms with predetermined dosing strategies. It is not essential to stick with a specific pattern of dosing, and it can vary according to personal needs and interests, which is not practice when it comes to western allopathic medicine.

Teas are made from the specific plants of the tea family, and leaves of tea plants are mostly used in this process. However, other parts, such as flowers, can also be used. It can be made from dried or fresh parts of tea making plants, and the servings per day can vary from 2-6 doses depending upon personal needs and tolerance. Sampling mixing the leaves of tea plants in a hot water cup and mixing with honey can provide thousands of health benefits, or it can be made by proper boiling and adding milk, etc. which is called actual fermentation of tea such as black tea.

Tea can be made from hand-picked leaves of tea plant grown in self botanic gardens, or it can be made from pre-designed herbal tea bags for convenience. When aromatic tea sources such as rosemary are used, its steam can also provide a face freshening treatment, which is a common practice in many western and Indian ayurvedic beauty treatments. Artificial or natural sweeteners such as honey can be used for adding more flavor to herbal teas. Stevia teas are naturally lovely in taste. Take a pinch of stevia tea, cool it in open-air then put it in a freezer bag. Then these bags can be put flat in freezers. When hit, a layer of frozen stevia tea can be break into ice chips, which can be used in other drinks to sweeten them as well as many benefits of stevia tea can be obtained through this process in regular drinks.

Decoctions

Decoctions are widely used sources of herbal medicine in herbalism. When roots or barks of plants contain medicinal benefits, it is hard to obtain extracts from these hard parts of plants, such as willow bark. Decoctions are great ways when the extraction of herbal medicine is required from these hard parts of plants. To obtain this, simmer the herb in hot water pan for at least twelve to thirty minutes on low flame. 1:32 ratio is essential to obtain decoctions from the herbs. A commonly used recipe involves 30 grams of herb and 1000ml of water.

Teas and decoctions are widely used as a herbal source of medicine preparation, and the reason behind using them on a wide-scale is easy to use properties. Just sipping through the cup is all it requires to administer the medicine inside the body. Even rinses and gargles can also be made from these two sources to relieve symptoms related to mouth and throat diseases.

Popsicles:

Popsicles can be made from a variety of sources, and it is an excellent source of reducing inflammation and pain related to the oral mucosa. Another benefit of popsicle is its incredible taste and ease of use.

Ice cubes:

Ice cubes are a fantastic source of herbal delivery, and they are straightforward to administer. It can be made from teas and decoctions as well. Liquid herbal medicine can be frozen after boiling and rapid cooling, a process called thawing. It also contains pain-relieving benefits, which are very specific with cold therapy. If we add sticks inside ice cubes, they can easily be turned into homemade sweet popsicles. This form of administration is highly famous among children. The ice bags and trays should be labeled accordingly to avoid issues.

Baths:

The largest organ of the body is skin, which has a very complicated structure and very diverse in properties and colors. Skin is porous and can allow transmission of medicine into deep structures when suitable media is used. Teas and decoctions are also used in bathing to enhance the delivery of medicine, for example, in sauna bathing. Hands and feet can be bathed alone in pots filled with herbal water, or full body can be soaked in a bathtub to achieve the medicinal benefits of herbal medicine. In bedridden patients, a damp cloth with medicinal fluid in it is a smart way of medicinal bed bathing. Hot baths are essential because they can make skin porous, and thus more drugs can be administered inside the body. Care should be taken when using a hot water bath to avoid burns and bruising. Bathing can be achieved by directly introducing dried herbs in bathtubs or pots to unlock maximum healing benefits. These herbs can be inserted directly in the bathtub, or these can be introduced in porous clothes like socks, pantyhose, and other delicate clothes to avoid a mess. Even loofa made from herbs can be used to be rubbed on the skin directly to maximize the absorption of the medicine through the skin. It is the smartest way of administration, but it can turn bathtubs a little messy and hard to clean.

Breast milk:

Infants can also use herbal medicine, but the route of administration, as well as dosing, can be very troublesome to decide. A full cup of tea and an ice cube of decoction is a terrible idea when used for infants. We have to decide the safest routes of administration because of the delicate body of infants. Breast milk is a natural source to nourish babies from the nutrients in the mother's blood. Breast milk is the safest from all the routes of nourishment because many complex nutrients that cannot be introduced in an infant's body otherwise can easily be inserted through breast milk. A mother and her child, both can be benefited in that way. Some herbal medicines are really infant friendly while others can be harsher on the delicate infant body, so a careful consideration before administration is essential to avoid any kind of side effects. Another significant benefit is to insert potent herbal antibacterial medicine inside an infant to make more him/her more immune with side effects of getting sick from antibacterials is to introduce them from the mother's breast milk. It will boost the natural immunization responses in both mother and her infant.

<u>Washcloths:</u>

Washcloths are indeed a great source to get bathed on the bed. They can be used on a critically ill patient who cannot survive an active bath. In this comfortable way, medicine can easily be applied to the skin, and thus it can be transferred in a deeper area of the body through diffusion. Washcloths can be warm by using hot infusions of medicine when specific impacts of heating are needed, or they can be cold when benefits of cold are needed. It all depends upon personal choice as well as symptoms of illnesses. For acute injuries, for example, brushing and combat sports fights, cold washcloths with specific benefits of ice and anti-inflammatory medicine can be a smart choice to limit swelling and bruising as well as impeding bleeding from fresh wounds. Cold also has anesthetic properties, which make it a natural pain killer.

When used warm, washcloths can stimulate blood flow due to vasodilatory effects as well as a soothing response of the body can also be obtained.

Compresses:

Compresses are warm medicinal pastes which are formed from many potent herbs. It is a very traditional technique, which is also caller "Marham" in Arabic, and it is the most used technique in Indian ayurvedic as well. Warm herbs in the form of compresses can stay longer than washcloths on the skin and can be a great source of constant delivery of herbal medicine. Feeling of warmth is soothing itself, and it also helps in reducing muscle spasm when applied. It also helps in vasodilation in specific areas to speed up recovery. Some herbs are delightful in fragrance and thus can provide the body with an unusual odor. Any natural fiber, a cloth with pores or muslin bag, can be used to form compresses from medicinal herbs. In traditional herbal medicine, compresses were formed by putting them in direct sunlight to get the effects of warmth. In modern days, ovens can be used to achieve the temperature and thus applied to the skin in comfortable ways. Microwaving should be avoided when other natural sources are available because of the health hazards of artificial heating. Different and multiple layers are also used over single compress to achieve maximum absorption as well as the mixing of herbs. It also protects from overheating and bruising.

Poultices:

Poultice or Marham is a type of herbal medicine that is applied to skin sores and wounds directly to achieve healing at maximum pace and to unlock bactericidal and anti-inflammatory benefits. It is an excellent source of delivering medicine from the skin to other, more profound layers of the body. Again, it is popular forms of medicine in traditional Chinese, Indian, and Muslim herbalism. It is so easy to apply the poultices that it can be applied to gums in mouth as well as on lips to treat symptoms of herpes and other STDs. Any type of fresh, damp, or dried herbs can be used to make poultices. Another effective way to apply them is to keep them on wounds for more extended periods to achieve maximum absorption. It is a widely used method of administration in herbal dentistry because it is by far the safest method to be used in the oral cavity. A poultice can be left overnight or longer in the mouth to avoid bruising and sores in the mouth. It will also help in improving the freshness of mouth and thus promoting the better odor in breath. It is essential to know the dosage of the herb in a poultice. A poultice is a damp or less wet type of medication, more like a paste which can be made by just mixing water, tea or decoction in a dried paste of herb. A mixture of different herbs can also be used to make a poultice to unlock many benefits hidden in these different herbs. It is a fantastic strategy that is used by many herbalists. For example, an analgesic herb containing pain killer properties can be mixed with antioxidant, anti-inflammatory, or any type of bactericidal herb to achieve all these impacts by a single use of poultice. A great recipe involves the use of herbal tea with blueberry along with willow to unlock the actions of all these three herbs in a single poultice.

Tinctures

Tinctures are drops of herbs in liquid form, which are combined in 80-95% of the alcohol base. The most crucial benefit of this type of administration is the very long preservation period of medicine achieved by adding alcohol into it. It is such a diluted form of medicine that hardly any side effect can occur. This is the sole reason that homeopaths used these types of tinctures from centuries to administer drugs in human bodies. The tincture can be prepared by mixing herb into wine, vodka, or rum. A more diluted media such as apple cider vinegar or glycerine can also be used to achieve these benefits. Alcohol-free media can also be used to make tinctures of very diluted quality for those who don't like alcohol to get ingested. Tinctures can be prepared in homes as well as they can also be available in markets. However, the best practice is to make it at home because it doesn't require any special treatment to prepare all these effective tinctures at home. Lany herbalists are famous for making their own tinctures. Raw alcohol is best to make tinctures rather than flavored vodka or rum so that the maximum benefits of herbs can be preserved. Flavoring is also rich in dirty surfers, which are not the right choice for medicinal purposes. Grain alcohol is the most popular type of alcohol used by herbalists to achieve the preparation of the highest quality tinctures. Vodka and grain are very different because they are made from very different sources. Twenty percent net alcohol should be used when the dried herb is made, and 40% of alcohol can be mixed with the fresh herb to ensure proper mixture and administration without side effects.

Willow bark is known to have high tannin concentration, and thus adding a few amounts of glycerin can be a smart idea for extracting maximum concentration of herb. A tincture is nothing when inferior ingredients are used. Alcohol is just a base in it; however, the medicinal benefits of a tincture can only be achieved from using proper herbs only. A perfect ratio is 1:5, that is 1 part alcohol with five parts of herbs to ensure more concentration of herb in a tincture. This guide is a critical ad accepted in herbalist society all over the world.

. In the case of yarrow, we make an alcohol-based. Yarrow or other types of tannin-containing herbs can be mixed with glycerine and alcohol to extract the medicinal benefits from them properly. The next stage is to put the solution in a dark room while keeping the solution in a tight jar for more than three weeks. A proper shaking the jar every week can also promote proper extraction of the herbal medicinal benefits.

The use of tea and decoction, along with water, can also be applied while making an alcohol free tincture. The final step of tincturing is to stain the solution. The solution is called menstruum, which, while stained, is called a tincture. It is essential to label the jar with the proper name for identification purposes.

These are common and most effective techniques to prepare proper herbal medications at home with much effort and preparation.

Summary:

His book is about the basics of medical herbalism for beginners. It consists of six chapters, and every chapter is dedicated to specific information which can be used to know all the hidden benefits of various herbs used in medical herbalism. It contains details about growing one's own medical herbs at home as well as many different ways of getting all the beneficial extracts from different herbs are also discussed. Traditional uses and specific histories, along with scientific evidence, are incorporated in this book to help in providing evidence-based guidelines about medical herbalism. The second series of this book will help in knowing the hidden secrets about medical herbalism against viral and infectious diseases.